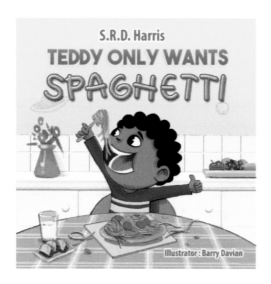

This book or parts thereof may not be reproduced in any form, stored in any retrieval system, or transmitted in any form by any means—electronic, mechanical, photocopy, recording, or otherwise—without prior written permission of the publisher, except as provided by United States of America copyright law. For permission requests, write to the publisher, at Attention: Permissions Coordinator via email at srdharrisbooks@gmail.com.
All rights reserved.

ISBN: 978-1-954674-00-4
Library of Congress Control Number: 2020925698
www.srdharrisbooks.com

Published by S.R.D. Harris Books, LLC and proudly printed in the USA.
Written by: S.R.D. Harris   Illustrated by: Barry Davian

D1223926

Teddy only wants spaghetti, much to his Mom's fright.
Teddy wants to eat spaghetti morning, noon, and night.

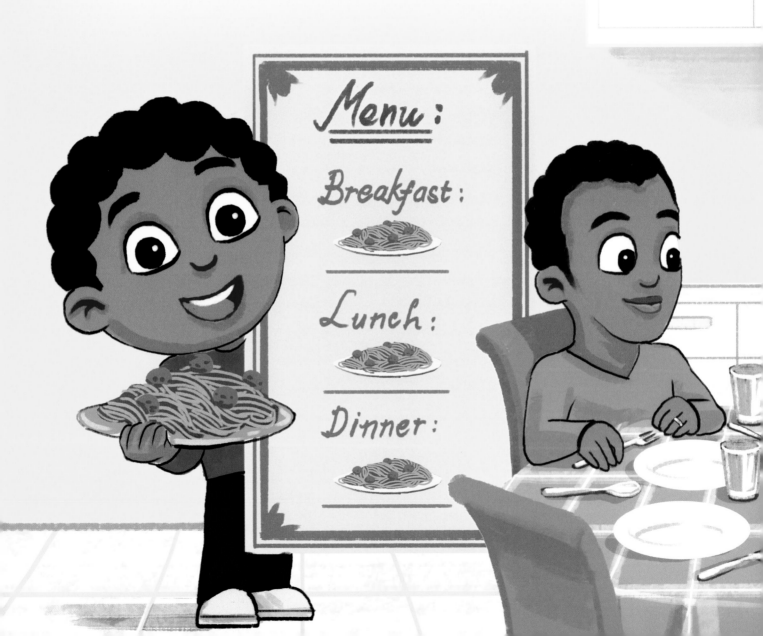

He always says "please" with manners in his voice.
Teddy thinks spaghetti is always the perfect choice.

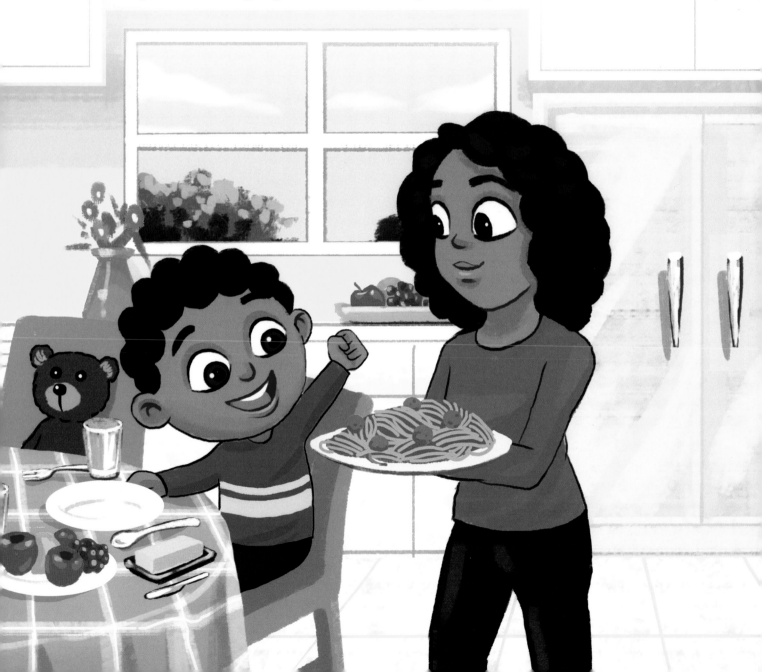

As soon as Teddy was old enough to learn how to cook.
He made his Mom's recipe, and didn't even need a cookbook.

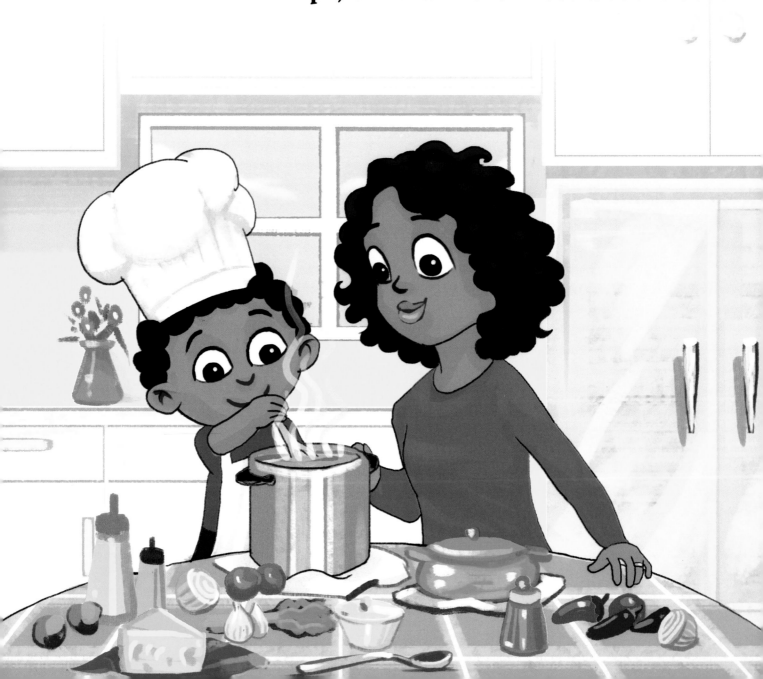

He always rolls his meatballs into the perfect spheres.
Teddy loves to make giant meatballs, bigger than elephant ears!

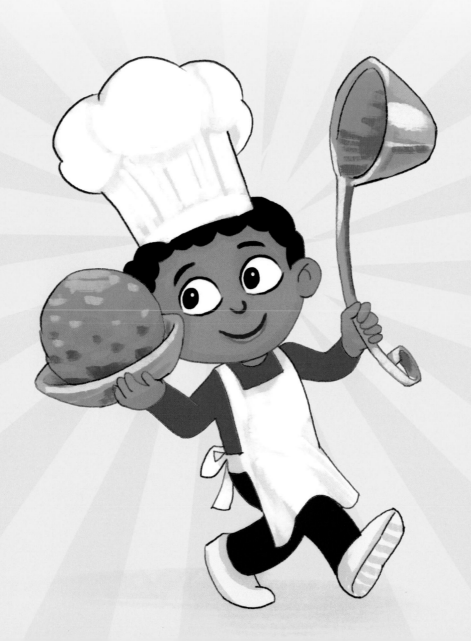

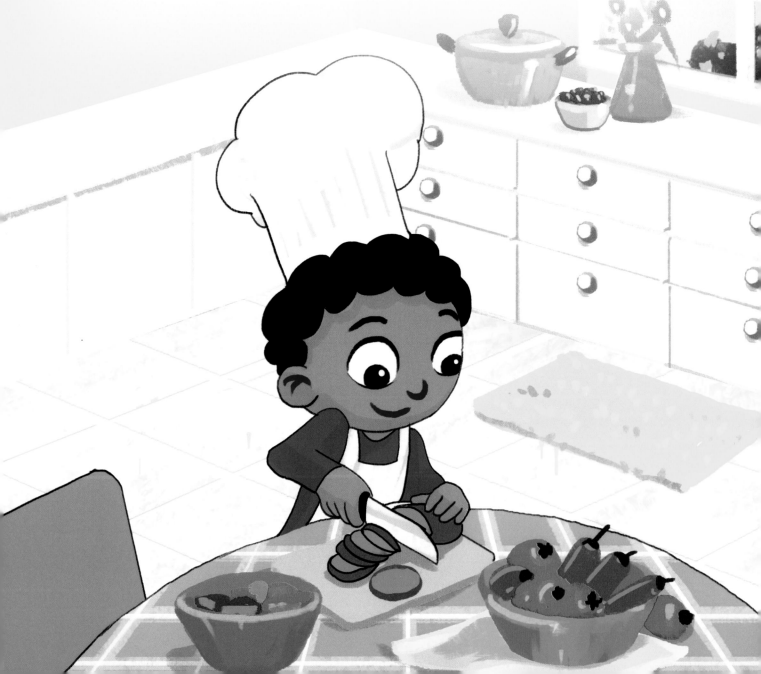

Teddy chops the peppers, tears the basil, and stirs the sauce around.
He piles the noodles on his plate in a great big giant mound!

He shreds some fresh parmesan and sprinkles it on top.
Spaghetti is his favorite food that he wants to eat nonstop!

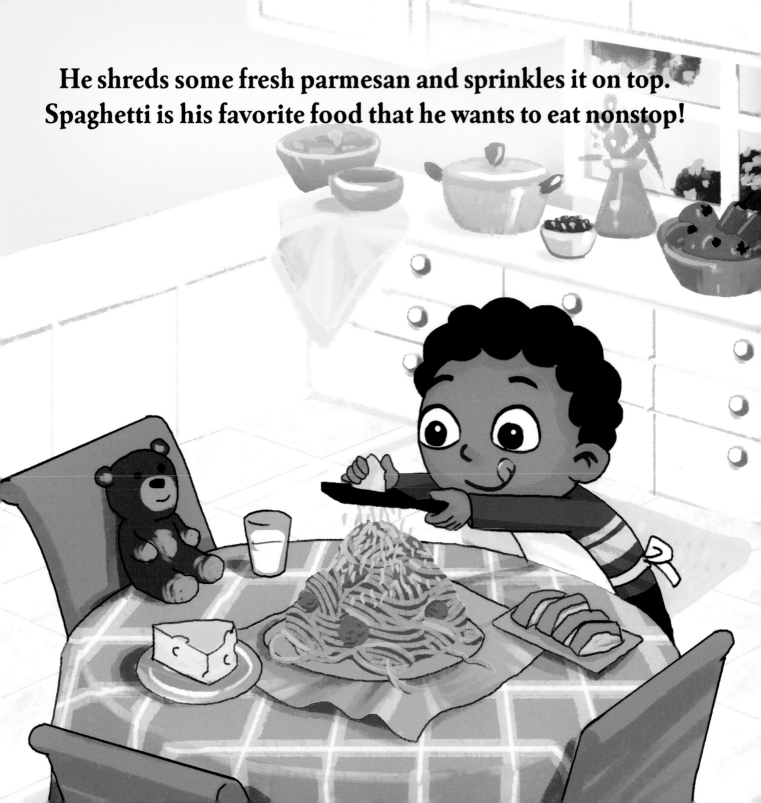

His Dad could cook a wonderful meal anyone would eat with ease.
But, once again, like always, Teddy asks "spaghetti please?"

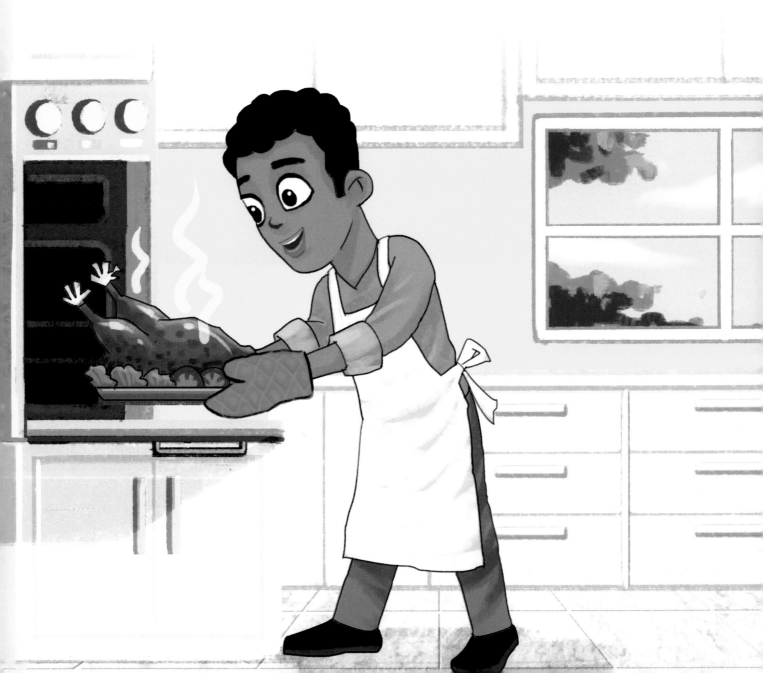

Dinner would be so much better if spaghetti is all we ate,
Teddy thought to himself as Dad put chicken on his plate.

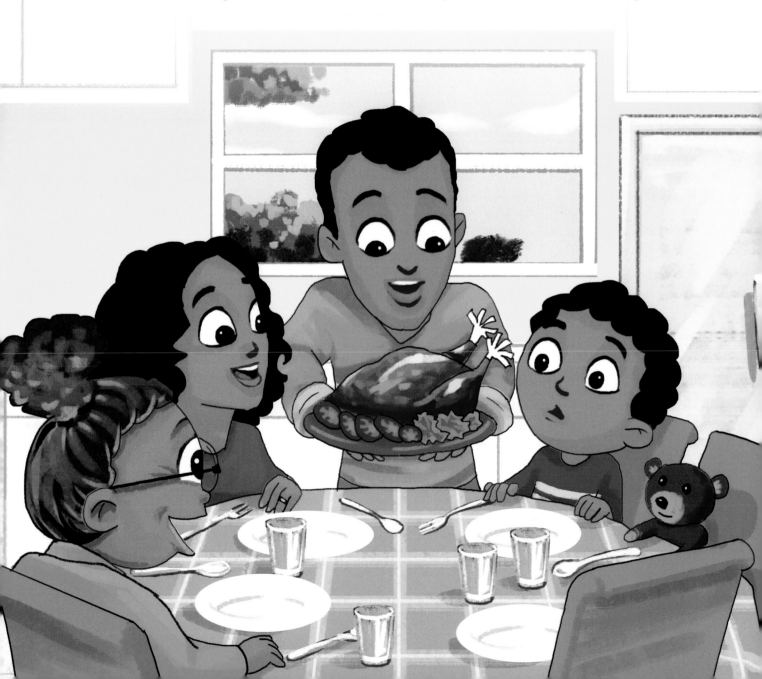

When his Gigi takes him out to dinner for his birthday treat.
She always knows just what Teddy will ask her to eat.

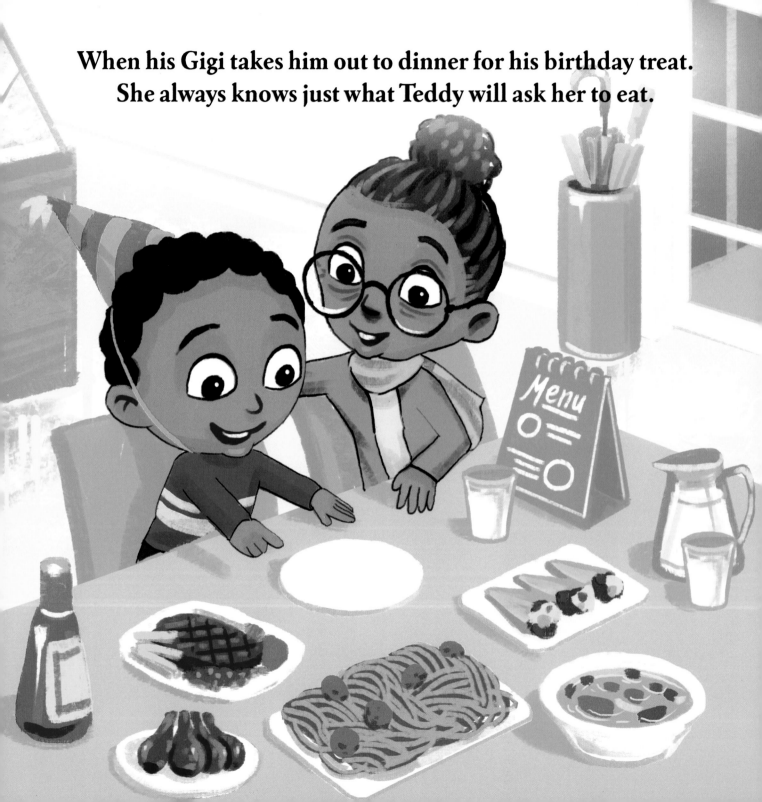

On his 8th birthday, Teddy made a very special wish.
"I wish I could be Spaghetti Boy, just like my favorite dish."

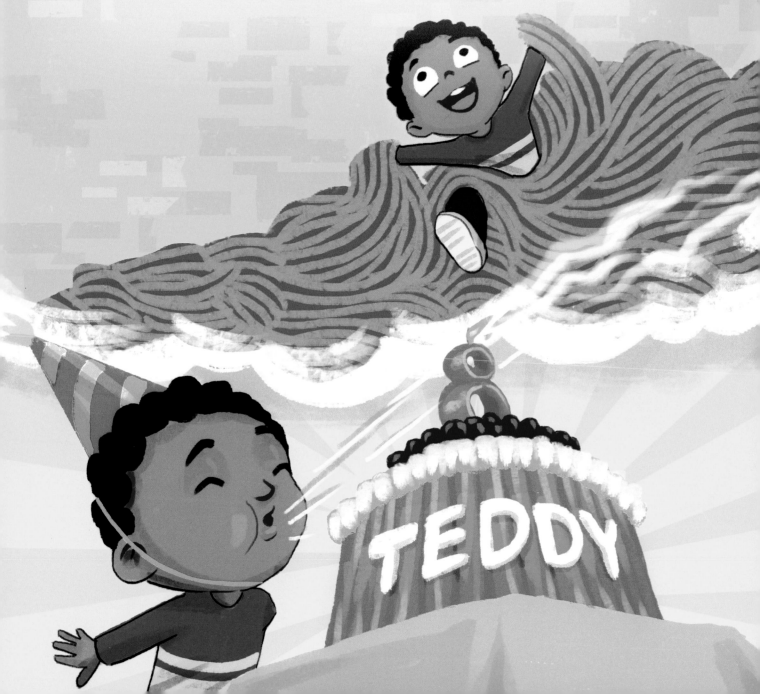

Teddy went to sleep that night dreaming of noodles and sauce.
But when he woke up the next morning, he felt a little off.

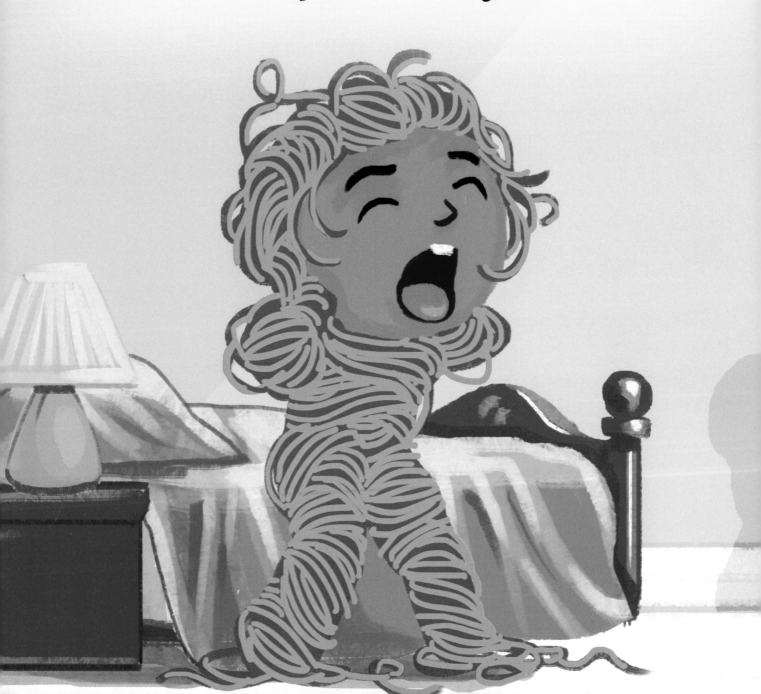

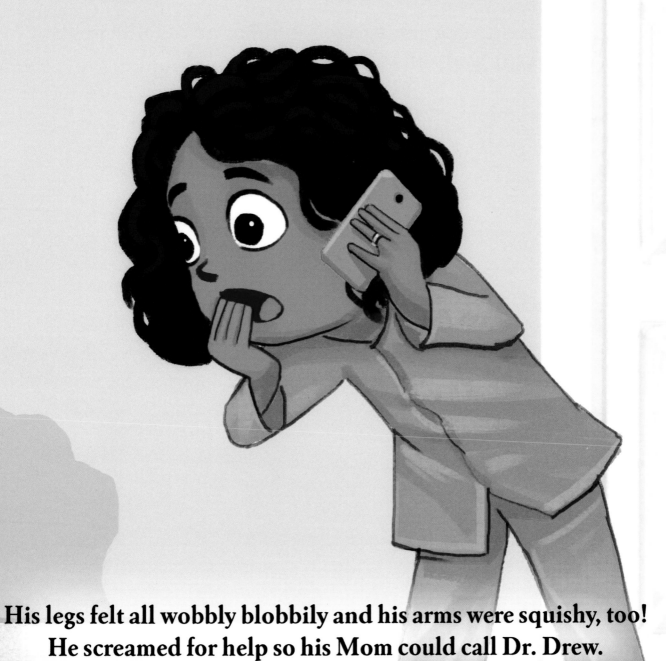

His legs felt all wobbly blobbily and his arms were squishy, too!
He screamed for help so his Mom could call Dr. Drew.

Mom said, "Teddy you can't go to school or go outside to play!"
"The birds and squirrel will eat you up with you looking that way!"

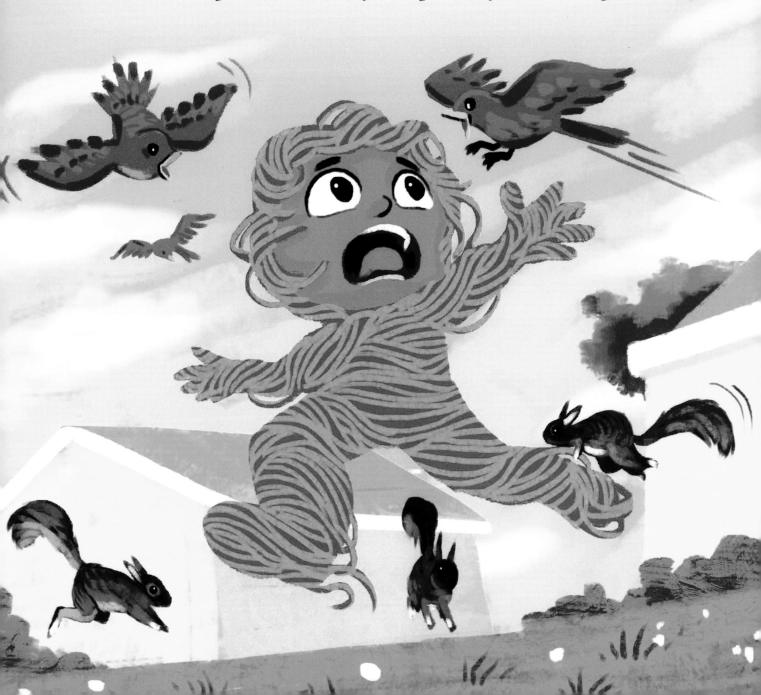

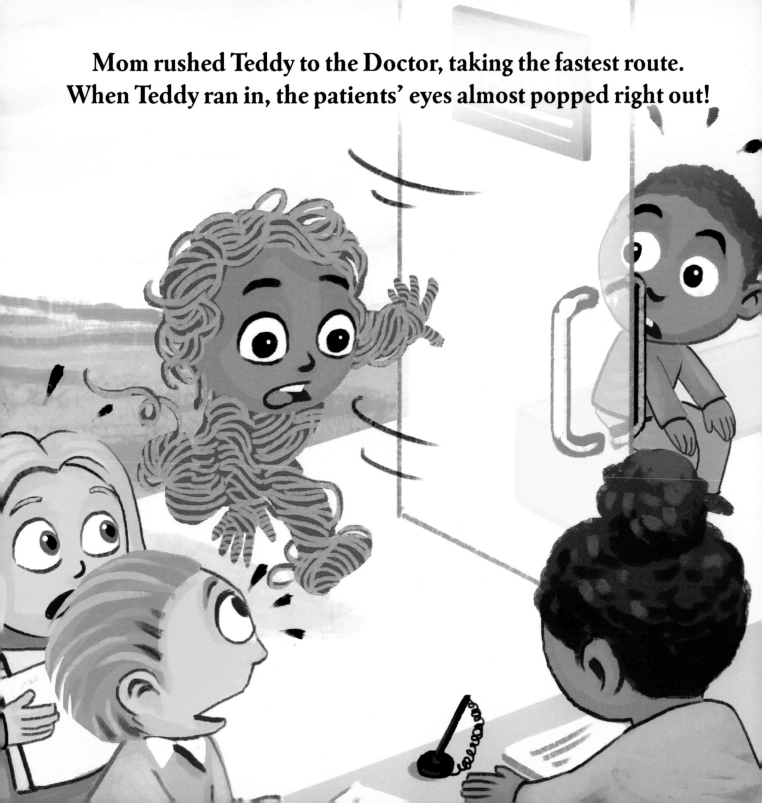

Mom rushed Teddy to the Doctor, taking the fastest route.
When Teddy ran in, the patients' eyes almost popped right out!

Dr. Drew checked Teddy out and knew exactly what to do.
"You have to start eating more foods, like fruits and veggies, too!"

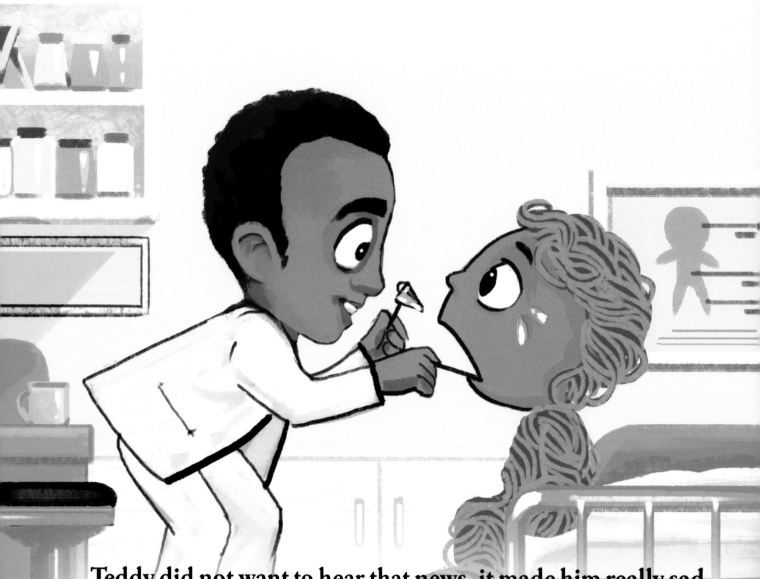

Teddy did not want to hear that news, it made him really sad.
But, he also knew getting eaten by birds would feel very bad.

Mom cooked him tasty meals, with fruits and veggies galore.
It was so good, Teddy didn't even miss spaghetti anymore.

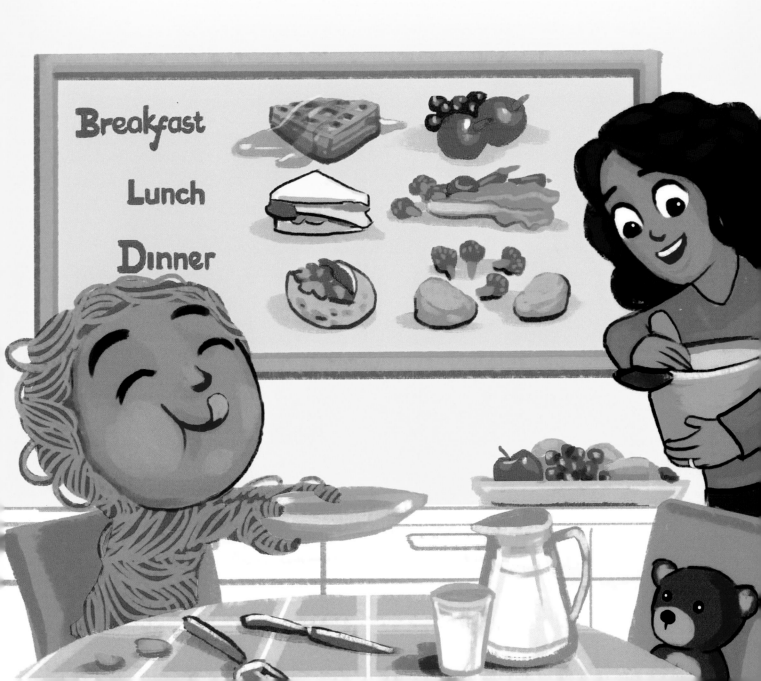

That night, Teddy skipped his bath and went straight to bed.
He quietly whispered another wish, and this is what he said.

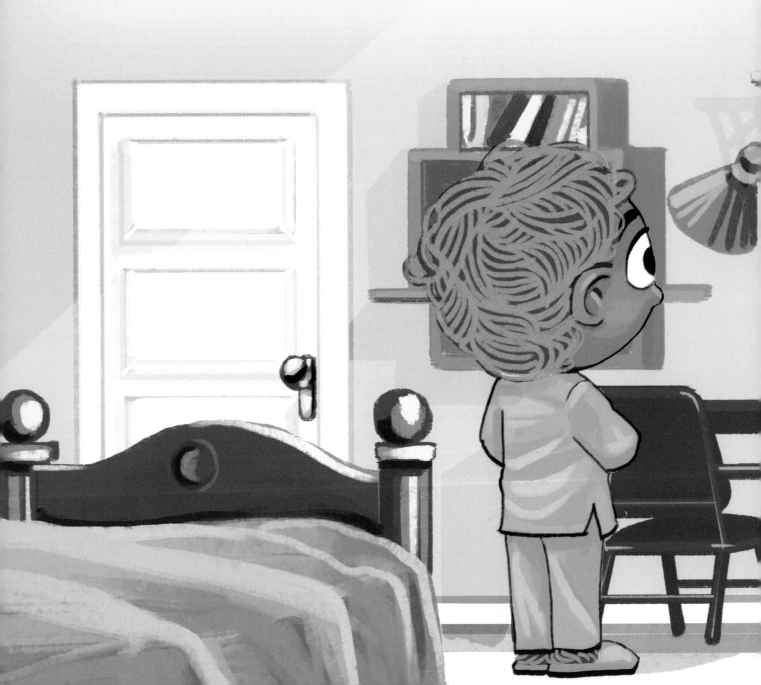

"I will always love spaghetti best, but I know what I must do.
I wish to be back to my old self, and not feel like globbily goo!"

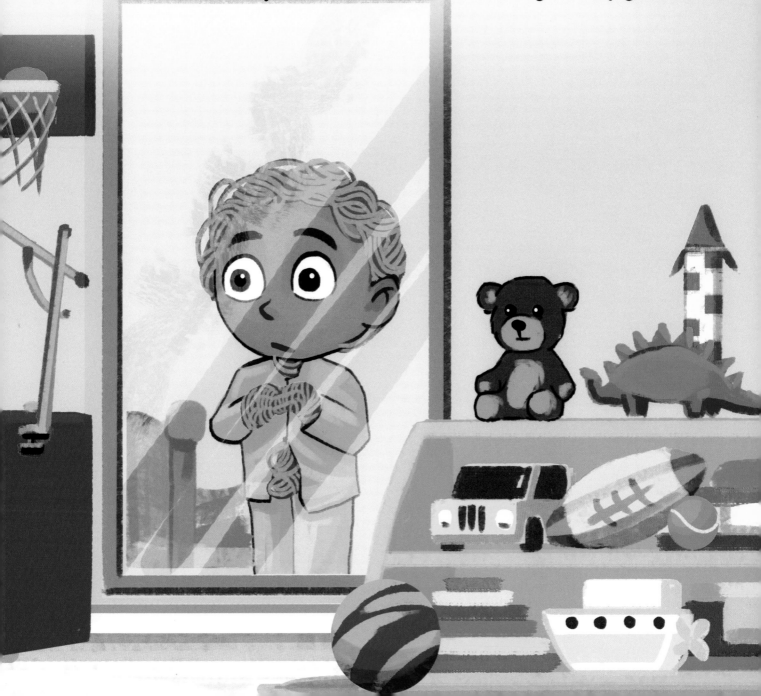

When Teddy woke up the next morning, he felt as good as new!
It was fun to be Spaghetti Boy, but he was glad that was through!

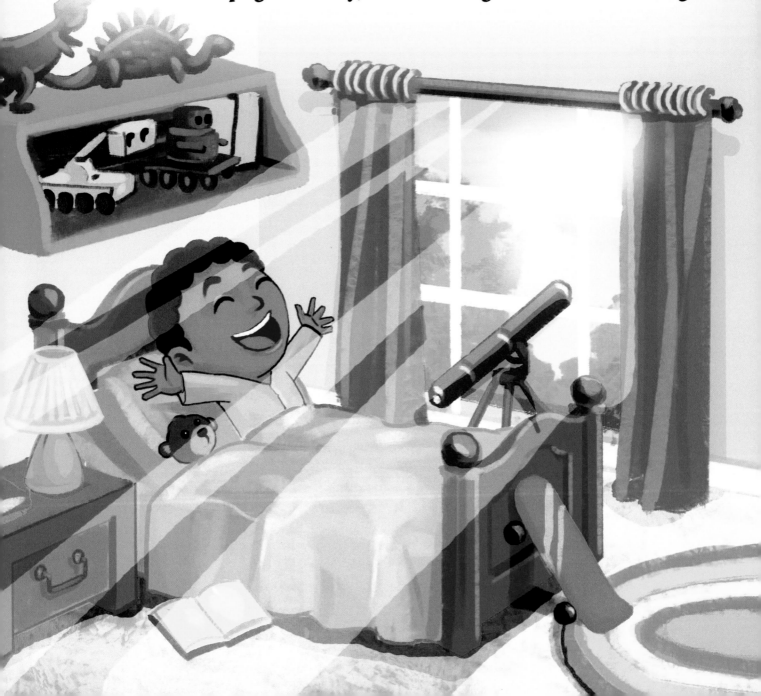

Teddy couldn't wait to get dressed and go outside to play!
Would his friends believe he was Spaghetti Boy yesterday?

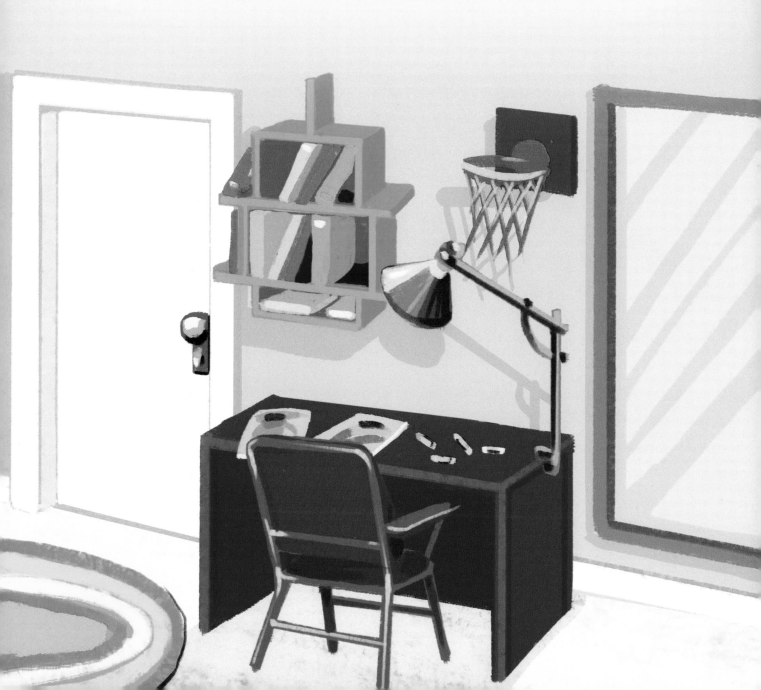

What important lesson did we learn from Teddy's story today?

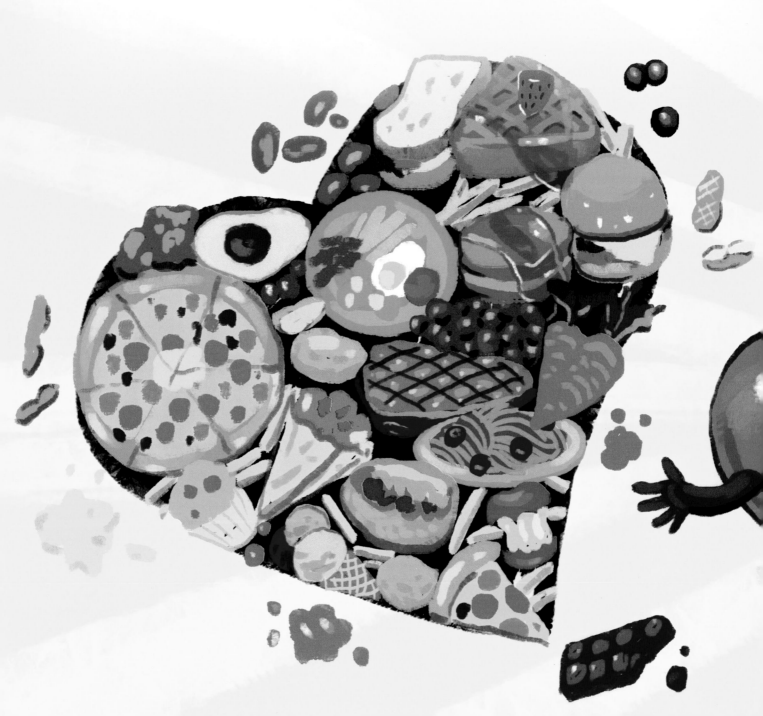

You are what you eat, so eat your fruits and veggies every day!

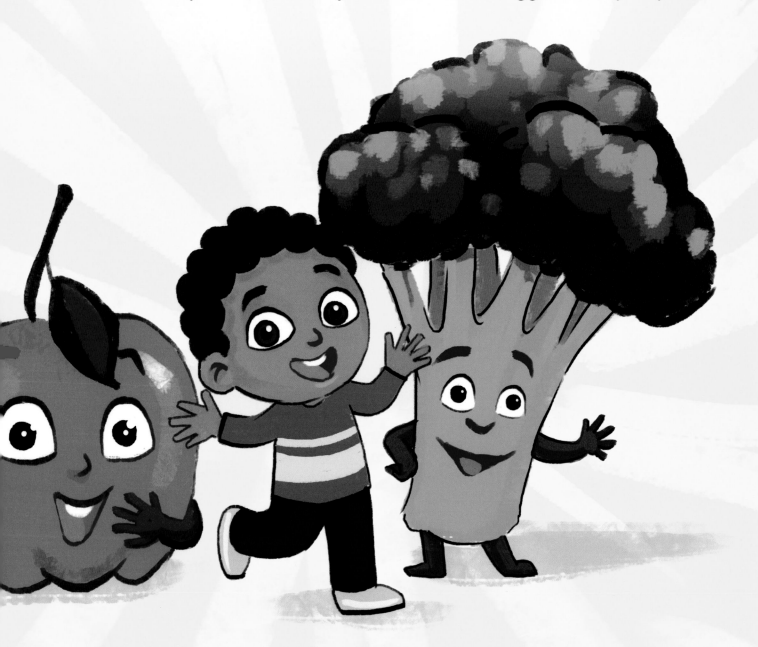

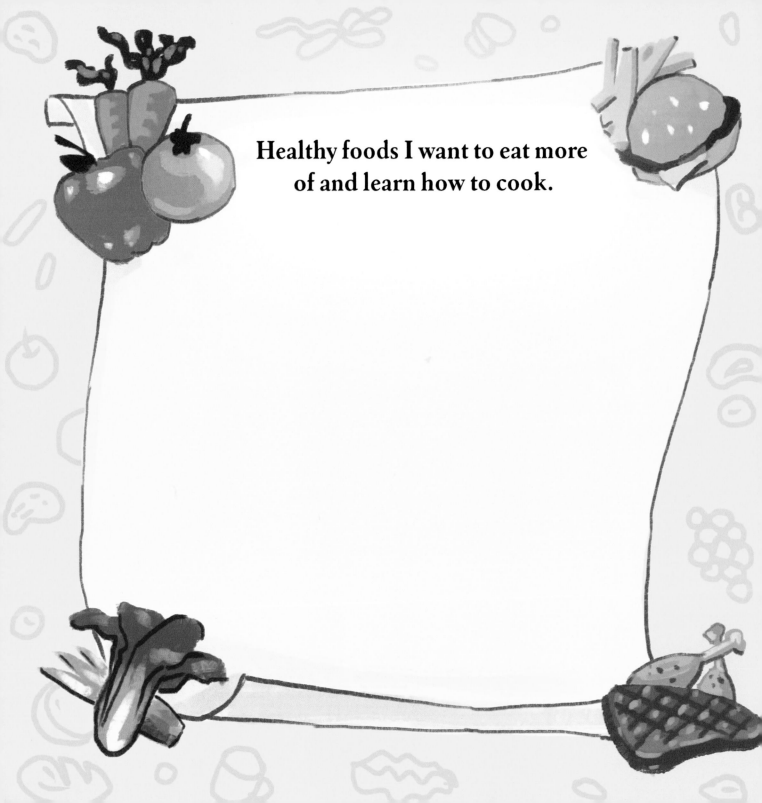

Healthy foods I want to eat more of and learn how to cook.

Thank You!

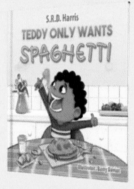

srdharrisbooks.com

This book is dedicated to my amazing husband
and our three wonderful daughters!
Thank you for your constant support, love, and encouragement!
Remember to always try new things and spice your life up with variety!

To readers and foodies everywhere---keep reading and trying new things!
To my wonderful friends and family, thank you for your tremendous support!

In loving memory of my first hero and best friend, my Daddy, T. E. Harris.